# Chemical Suicide

I0102311

Alika Hickman

## Alika Publishing Co.

ISBN-13: 9780615232904
ISBN-10: 0615232906
Revised first Printing

# Acknowledgements

I am very thankful to the following individuals and organizations who extended me permission to make liberal use of the contents of their writings and websites. Without which, I would have been unable to produce this book. Those individuals are as follows:

Lori Stryker
Rebecca Sutton
Anita Grant
Marianne
Stacy Malkan
Health Care Without Harm
Environmental Working Group

A more detailed statement of the works of those that I relied upon is stated in the credits section of this book.

Thank you to my left hand, because this whole book was created and typed by you.

To my Creator, Thank you for reminding me that all things are possible.

To my son Javon, you are truly my inspiration. Thank you for your wonderful spirit! This book is dedicated to you.

To my awesome mom, I love you dearly & thanks for believing in me.

To Mario Marshall, you are a great friend, and a great graphic master. I am grateful for your presence in my life.

# Chemical Suicide

## Introduction

Like most people, "I have been a Cosmetic, and Household Cleaner Junkie!" I would wash my hair with a great sudsy shampoo, and then condition it with a recommended conditioner that seemed to work. Then I would stick to that brand until slowly but surely the brand started deceiving me. My hair would start drying out and breaking off badly, for no apparent reason. Being the African American woman that I am, my first instinct was to go purchase grease, and grease my scalp. On other occasions, I would go to my beautician and get a deep conditioner or whatever else recommended to fix the problem.

On April 9$^{th}$ of 2007 due to a 2nd aneurysm in the brain, I was rushed to the hospital. While undergoing surgery I had a stroke. When I came to, I was paralyzed on my right side and I couldn't speak. The physicians informed my family the likelihood is that I would never walk or talk again. After going through a dramatic brain surgery and having my hair completely shaved off, I was told that I could not put any chemicals on my hair for at least a year or so. I was very confused about what I should do with my hair in the meantime. After all, I had been using chemicals in my

1

hair since I was twelve years old. My immediate decision was to let my hair grow out long enough to attach braided hair extensions to it. Over a period of time, I became tired of wearing the braids and decided to wear my natural hair.

After becoming a natural sister, I went to my local beauty supply store and bought a dye that made my hair a luminous blonde which in turn made my hair feel dry, brittle, and also caused it to break excessively. Once again I went to the beauty supply and bought some hair grease and greased it up! It was at this point of complete disgust that I started searching the internet for information on how I could keep my natural hair healthy without using the concoctions of greases and chemicals that I had used since I was twelve years old. Finally, I found out some very disturbing information: I AM NOT SUPPOSED TO USE GREASE ON MY HAIR OR SCALP! What!?! I have been using grease all my life, and my hair has grown. "I think." Yes my hair has grown with grease. However, the information I read indicated that grease is unnecessary because the scalp produces its own oil (sebum) that naturally moisturizes the scalp. The petroleum in the hair grease clogs up the pours of the scalp and blocks the oils that our scalps naturally produce. Likewise, mineral oil and petroleum, which are extensively used in most hair products, are also in the same family with gasoline.

Continuing my search, I discovered how mineral oil and petroleum are bad for your skin because they also clog the pores and don't allow the natural toxins of our bodies to be released, thus creating more problems internally. I have never really been an ingredients reader, however I have discovered that reading the ingredients is essential to understand what we are using on our bodies as well as in our bodies.

Frankly, I never understood the scientific wording of what is contained in the various products that we purchase for our bodies, for example; Sodium laurel Sulfate, what is that? I, like most people bought the products because they were advertised to fix those things that we felt would help us look and feel better. But I look on the back of my hair grease, and the first ingredient is petrolatum, second ingredient mineral oil. Then I go to both the shampoo and the conditioner, and they contain the same ingredients, plus the Sodium laurel sulfate. So my next search was to find out what sodium laurel sulfate is. What I found was mind blowing!

I found out that Sodium laurel sulfate is detergent and or surfactant used in car wash soaps, garage floor cleaners, engine and sink degreasers, cosmetics, toothpaste, and over

90% of all shampoos and products that foam. Animals exposed to SLS(sodium laurel sulfate) experienced eye damage, depression, labored breathing, diarrhea, skin irritation, and even death! Wow! If it can cause all these problems in animals, one can only imagine what it does to human beings. I was just your typical black girl going "back to" natural, and I have discovered a world of chemicals that may be assisting me and you to an early grave. While SLS, Mineral Oil, and Petrolatum's are some of the main harmful chemicals in most beauty products that I have mentioned, there are hundreds more that are equally damaging to the human body.

My main mission for this book is to enlighten those of us who are not familiar with the sources of damages that we are doing to ourselves. Most of us are misinformed about the dangerous toxins that we are using to make ourselves more *beautiful.* We have turned the cosmetic companies into a multi million dollar industry, while the chemicals in these products are linking us to cancer, brain hemorrhages, skin diseases, birth defects, contamination, skin lesions, and early aging. And to top it all off, the FDA does not require that cosmetic companies include a list of the ingredients that were chosen to make the product. I guess they figured we would purchase it anyway. And they are right.

I have included the definitions of over 20 toxins that are found in your Shampoos, Conditioners, lipstick, perfume, deodorants, foundations, lotions, sunscreens, anti aging, face creams, etc.

On the other hand I have provided you with homemade beauty recipes to make most of the products listed above. Most of the homemade recipes can be made right in your kitchen! I will also give you a list of natural ingredients that you can use. For example, if the ingredients for a recipe says add avocado, you can try adding banana as well, GET CREATIVE! That's the thing with homemade recipes, you don't have to make it just one-way, just make it so it fits you. I have also included blank pages for you to keep track of what ingredients you have added, or subtracted from your recipes. For example, when making the perfumes, what essential oils you decided to mix, and what amounts. You can also use the blank sheets to record the content of your recipes.

And remember, you are the consumer. If you don't like it, don't buy it. Become a label reader. And anything that looks suspicious, find out the meaning.

## Petroleum and Cosmetics: What are the Potential Health Risks?

What is petroleum?

Crude oil, sometimes called petroleum, is a fossil fuel that was produced deep in the earth through a process that took millions of years to complete.

Millions of years later, almost all of us come into contact with a derivative of petroleum every day. Through a process called fractional distillation, petroleum refineries break petroleum into many of its smaller components. Each of these smaller components is made up of molecules called hydrocarbons.

The world is full of products that come from petroleum. For example, **gasoline, styrofoam, lubricating oils**, and many other items are all derivatives of this raw material. How are petroleum and cosmetics related? The two seemingly unrelated items, petroleum and cosmetics, are indeed closely related in our modern world.

Mineral oil and petroleum are the basic ingredients in many cosmetic products today. Both mineral oil and petroleum have the same origins in fossils fuels. Cosmetics such as foundations, cleansers, and moisturizers often contain mineral oil. By locking moisture against the skin, mineral oil sits on the skin's surface and can potentially block pores. This may cause the appearance of pimples because the skin cannot properly "breathe".

Fragrances in **lotions, shampoos**, and many other cosmetic products are composed of aromatic hydrocarbons. Perfumes and products containing fragrance can contain many hundreds of chemicals to produce a distinct scent. A significant number of these aromas are derived from petroleum.

One popular chemical additive that carries moisture in cosmetics is propylene glycol. It is also a derivative of petroleum. Some products that list propylene glycol as an ingredient include:

- Anti-freeze

- Laundry detergent

- Paint

- Shampoo

- Conditioner

Past research links propylene glycol to serious health problems such as liver and kidney damage as well as respiratory irritation or nausea if swallowed.

An antiseptic, isopropyl alcohol, kills bacteria on the skin. You can find it on the ingredient list of cleansers, toners and other cosmetic products. Unfortunately, this derivative of petroleum dries the skin and may cause miniature cracks in the skin that allow bacteria to enter, potentially causing irritations or pimples.

Do these petroleum-derived products affect your health?

Your skin covers your body and acts as a physical barrier to many of the pollutants in the atmosphere. When you use products on your skin such as cosmetics, lotions, and shampoos, the ingredients in these products come into direct contact with your body's largest organ; your skin. You may ask yourself, where do the ingredients in the products go? Modern research at the Herb Research Foundation found that the skin absorbs up to 60% of the chemicals in products that it comes into contact with directly into the bloodstream. Today, hormone therapy treatments and smoking cessation medications are often prescribed as patches that you apply directly to the skin.

The medication passes through the skin and directly enters the bloodstream.

For pregnant women, the risk is not only for her body but also for the developing fetus. If the chemicals found in cosmetics readily enter the bloodstream when applied to the skin, then they will also reach the developing baby. Researchers at the Brunel University in England are looking closely at a family of preservatives called parabens. Their research has recently linked parabens to the possibility that male babies will have lower sperm counts. These preservatives are derived from petroleum and help to maintain the freshness and integrity of the product. Currently, many manufacturers add parabens to cosmetics to allow a minimum of 3 years shelf life. Therefore, the parabens kill any bacteria that could potentially enter the product. If these chemical ingredients can kill the bacterial cells, what are they doing to your skin cells? In most cases, there is no conclusive answer to this question. However, the research mentioned strongly suggests that the synthetic ingredients may have a significant impact on our bodies.

In many cases, the long-term effects of many of the chemical additives in our cosmetics are not known. However, other chemical additives are known carcinogens. These types of chemicals can cause cancer in humans. Such chemicals include some artificial colors in cosmetics. The effects of chemicals and other synthetic ingredients in cosmetics may lead to mild allergic reactions causing rashes and minor skin irritation to more significant problems such as lesions on the skin.

**What are your alternatives for cosmetics?**

Luckily, there alternatives to cosmetics filled with synthetically produced ingredients. Increasingly, cosmetic manufacturers are answering the public's demand for alternatives to the chemically loaded beauty and grooming supplies. There are many companies that are producing chemical free beauty products. As a consumer, you have the ability to decrease the number of preservatives and chemical additives your skin comes into contact with and therefore, that may enter your body. To avoid using the synthetically derived fragrances, look for products containing essential oils. These are pure oils derived from flowers and other plants in nature.

All you have to do is make the simple choice of purchasing cosmetic products with all-natural, organic ingredients. Whether you continue using cosmetics that contain petroleum-based ingredients or not is a personal choice. What is the most important is to get the facts and to know that you have a choice when it comes to buying organic or synthetic cosmetic products.

Look on the back of your hair grease/oil/products and read what the ingredients are. Let me guess, first one is petrolatum/petroleum, second is mineral oil? Wow!

## Why Switch to All Natural Cosmetics?

The human skin wraps and protects our bodies. It constitutes a living, dynamic tissue system. It has the remarkable ability to absorb applied products, partially or completely, into the bloodstream. In fact, up to 60% of the products we use on our skin are absorbed and deposited into the circulatory system (*Fairley, 2001*). For instance, the average woman absorbs 30 pounds of the ingredients contained in moisturizers over sixty years (*Dr.Hauschka*).

These new understandings of how the skin functions reveal concerns about the possible long-term effects due to the combination of chemicals used in cosmetics, often termed the "chemical cocktail effect". Several chemicals, which are used, in common, popular cosmetics are known irritants and carcinogens. Concern stems from the knowledge that most of these ingredients are derived synthetically or from petroleum. Avoiding these substances serve to decrease overall exposure to harmful or irritating cosmetic ingredients.

The following chart contains a listing of substances found in beauty and grooming products and possible side effects. These products should not be used.

| Ingredients to Avoid | Forms Found in Cosmetics and Possible Negative Side Effects |
|---|---|
| Aluminum | Thought to contribute to Alzheimer's Disease. Found in almost all antiperspirants. Works by blocking pores so sweat cannot be released by the skin. |

| | |
|---|---|
| Artificial colors | FD&C, derived from coal tar. For example, Azo dyes are a risk to asthmatics, eczema sufferers and people sensitive to aspirin. Causes hyperactivity in children, severe headaches, blurred vision and itchy/watery eyes and nose (*Antczak, 2001*). |
| Benzoates | Benzoates Benzoic acid, sodium benzoate or parahydroxy benzoate. Used as a preservative in cosmetics and fizzy drinks. Causes gastric irritation, numbing of the mouth and aggravates asthma (*Antczak, 2001*). |

| Certain essential oils | Rosemary is harmful to epileptics. Sage is not recommended for pregnant women. |
| DEA, MEA, TEA | Causes allergic reactions, irritating to eyes and dries out hair and skin (*Fairley, 2001*). |

| Dibutyl phthalate | Found in all persons tested by the CDC (*Center for Disease Control, USA*) in a 2000 Fall study. Highest levels were found in women of reproductive age. Causes birth defects in animals, and damaging to the male reproductive system (*ABC News, Internet Ventures 2000*). Used in cosmetics to assist the absorption of other ingredients. |

| Formaldehydes | A preservative. Causes skin reactions. Imidazolidinyl urea is the second most identified preservative causing contact dermatitis ( *American Academy of Dermatology: Fairley, 2001*). |
| --- | --- |
| Other names for formaldehydes: DMDM Hydantoin Quaternium 15 Diazolidinylurea 2-bromo-2 nitropropane-1 3-diol | |

| | |
|---|---|
| Fragrances | Can contain up to 200 undeclared substances (*Fairley, 2001*). Major cause, in addition to artificial colors, of skin irritations and allergies (*Antczak, 2001*). May cause dizziness, skin irritation and hyper pigmentation (*Fairley, 2001*). |
| Genetically Modified Organisms | Human health effects of consuming GMO foods can include toxic and allergic reactions, antibiotic resistance, immune suppression, and other serious illnesses. |
| Isopropyl Alcohol | Drying agent, from petroleum. |

| Keratolytic chemicals | Such as hydroxyl acids, retinoic acid. Corrosive, used in skin peels. Dissolves the stratum corneum of the epidermis (*outermost layer*), making skin more sensitive to sun damage. Accelerates production of dead skin cells; the skin thickens to repair its surface so that vulnerable skin cells underneath are protected from the effects of skin peeling. (*Antczak, 2001*). |
|---|---|
| Methylisothiazolinone | Causes allergic reactions and irritations (*Fairley, 2001*). |

| | |
|---|---|
| Parabens | Petroleum product. Triggers skin irritations and may be an xerestrogen (*Fairley, 2001*).May play a role in falling sperm counts and rising breast cancer rates (Fairley, 2001).Used in 99% of all cosmetics (*Fairley, 2001*), and in many so-called *'natural'* products. |
| Paraffin | Derived from petroleum. In the form of wax, mineral oil or petrolatum. Comedogenic, i.e. blocks pores. |

| | |
|---|---|
| Propylene Glycol | When derived from petroleum. Increases the amount of acid in the body, resulting in metabolic problems. Large amounts are needed to produce this effect (*Agency for Toxic Substances and Disease Registry or ATSDR, 2003*). |
| Sodium laureth sulfate, sodium lauryl sulfate | Forms carcinogenic nitrogen compounds when combined with specific ingredients. Irritating to eyes, skin and lungs (*Antczak, 2001*). Harmful if swallowed and may cause damage to eyes (*Antczak, 2001*). |

| Tallow | Animal fat. Not suitable for vegans, and may be a skin irritant. |

| Toluene | Found in many nail products and nail polish removers. Produced during the process of making gasoline and other fuels from crude oil or coal. Evaporates into the air when products containing toluene are opened. May affect the nervous system, and/or cause tiredness, confusion, weakness, nausea, or loss of appetite. Symptoms disappear when exposure is eliminated (*ATSDR, 2003*). |

In Canada, not all cosmetics list their ingredients on their labels, but most have toll free telephone numbers which link you to their customer service departments, where inquiries about ingredient lists can be made. Reading labels and recognizing problematic ingredients are necessary skills for a consumer who intends to choose products that are completely natural. The cost of a cosmetic is not a reliable indicator of either its quality or natural characteristics. Most cosmetics, from the lowest priced, to the most costly brands, are composed of identical base ingredients (*Begoun, 1991*).

Cosmetics do not stay on the surface of the skin without penetrating it to some degree. Lipstick wearers, for example, consume 1.5 to 4 tubes in a lifetime (*Aveda*). If one considers the ingredients being internalized by the body, absorbing plant oils and waxes, mineral pigments or essential oils is a healthier alternative than absorbing petroleum by-products and synthetic chemicals.

The ability to choose the right cosmetics for you depends on accurate ingredient knowledge, personal needs and market choices. Caring for one's whole body includes skin care choices that support and contribute to a healthy lifestyle.

Natural cosmetic products and make-up are safer, healthier alternatives especially when these products are composed of all natural ingredients. A natural product is described as one that contains mostly or completely naturally derived ingredients (*Antczak, 2001*). It also indicates that the product is free from, or contains minute amounts of artificial chemical additives. Caution is required when products claim to be natural. For instance, they may contain small amounts of plant extracts, but the bulk of the product is petroleum based and loaded with fragrances. Instead, consider switching to completely natural products, which perform to the same standard as their non-natural counterparts.

Switching to all-natural cosmetic products and make-up can help you to avoid feeding your skin harmful chemicals. Many skin problems, such as acne, contact dermatitis, irritations and allergies may disappear once petroleum or synthetic ingredients are removed from your skin care regimen. Using fully natural products can contribute to healthy skin and a healthy body in the long term.

## Afro-American Women

In today's society, all women are feeling more pressure about being "Television Beautiful." We want to be exactly as the images are that we see on TV on a daily basis. The reality is those images are unrealistic to most African American women. I remember as a child, I would see black children that had a wavier pattern hair texture. And I remember adults around me saying "She has Good hair." Verses someone else who's' hair was kinkier (nappy) and it would be the opposite "That girl's hair is nappy, she needs a perm!"

Now, you don't have to be a rocket scientist to figure this out. If Black women are being told that they don't have "Good Hair" then without much thought, the immediate thought response is "My hair is *bad*." So now we are growing up with a complex about our "nappy/not good" hair. Psychologically we believe that we are ugly with our natural hair, so we must straighten it with a perm (Chemicals), make it shine with petroleum based products (chemicals), and continue this cycle of torture all in the name of "Beauty" as we see it.

When I first saw Erykah Badu, I was totally amazed at her presence. Her songs were amazing, but it was more her style, and her obviously natural beauty. This was definitely when I was a **perm**aholic. She was just so pretty to me, and now I know why I was so attracted to her, as well as Lauryn Hill; it was because they were Napptually Black and Beautiful.

Now I'm not saying "Everybody go cut the perm out and go kinky." But I am saying, look in the mirror and ask yourself, "How would I look with my natural hair?" If your answer is UGLY, or anything close to that, then you may want to do some soul searching.
Your reality is, your hair is naturally kinky-curly, and Kinky-Curly is beautiful. Black Women are Beautiful. And we are still beautiful with a perm, but the side-effects of perms is that over time, you are continuously putting chemicals on your scalp that are going into your bloodstream, linking you to breast tumors(parabens), and slowly threatening your life.

Now, I was one of those women that really had to have a perm. When I see would see new growth, then its time for the relaxer, which was not relaxing at all. And the thought of wearing my kinky hair was disgusting! If I did wear it kinky, how would I comb it? I am the most tender headed person ever!

Well, I learned that you can't comb Kinky hair the same way you do permed hair. When kinky hair is dry, unless it is pressed out, *don't Comb It,* or it will hurt. Our hair loves moisture, and water! You should condition it after washing it, but you can wet kinky hair every other day as long as you have a leave in conditioner (organic of course).

Oil does not work as a moisturizer; it just seals in the moisture. My suggestion is to get a good moisturizing conditioner (Organic), and use that, or use one of the homemade ones that have been suggested in this book.

There are lots of hairstyles that you can do with kinky hair. And if you want it straight, then press it. If you are in the process of transitioning from processed hair to natural there are several things you can do. You can always get braid extensions, or you can get a sew in weave that matches the texture of your natural hair until it grows to the length you desire.

I recently went to an online website called Anitagrant.com. The website advertised all natural products. This is what Anita Grant had to say about taking care of your kinky hair:

## KEEP YOUR SCALP MOIST:

To regulate the amount of sebum your scalp produces we suggest using/massaging it with Organic Watermelon Oil twice a month or using it as pre-shampoo oil. Watermelon oil is easily absorbed, dissolves excess sebum & adds a rich shine to the hair. If you use heavy hair care "grease" that contains petroleum by products, you may be preventing the production of sebum, which, inevitably leads to serious build up.

If your hair and/or scalp are **not** oil and/or butter friendly then use an herbal infusion. Select herbs that are packed full of plant protein.

## BUILD UP:

Build up is inevitable because we, as humans, secrete sebum and sweat from the apocrine (sweat) glands and sebaceous glands located in the dermal layer (second layer) of our skin/scalp. At the same time when our old skin/scalp tissue cells regenerate and sloths off naturally as dead skin/scalp tissue new skin/scalp tissue forms.

Everybody is different but if you have an overactive gland or two, which is covered by a heavy chemical petroleum grease, then the dead skin cells lining the opening of you hair follicle will not shed properly and clog up your hair follicles - producing build up - which creates an ideal environment for bacteria. Bacteria loves heavy oils that are not easily absorbed into the skin.

### *BUILD UP "MAY NOT BE" PRODUCT RELATED:*

Regardless of which product you use you may be prone to build up because of your glands plus the slothing off of dead skin/scalp cells and not the product(s) you use. This is why it is always best to clarify your hair and scalp at least once a week (either with an ACV (apple cider vinegar) mix or Baking Soda + Water mix or herbs + ACV or 100% pure unsweetened Apple Juice or add baking soda to your shampoo).

### Coloring

Coloring with permanent hair dye causes damage to the chemical structure of the hair cuticle.
Blow dryers are a potential danger to hair, especially if your hair is chemically treated as it alters the protein bonds that hold the

hair together. With the application of heat you are in effect breaking those bonds, causing the ends of your hair to split all the way up the hair shaft.
The only way to repair it is to get the damaged hair trimmed or cut and start over.

If you were to use the blow dryer on your skin in exactly the same way you use it on your hair you will damage your skin as it will become dry, itchy and flaky.

## What curly & wavy hair doesn't need:

Anita Grant's opinion: curly-coily, wavy hair (regardless of ethnicity) should not be exposed to harsh drying methods and/or harsh ingredients like:
 SLS (Sodium Lauryl Sulphate)
 Dimethicone - Silicone
 Cyclomethicone - Silicone
 Propylene Glycol - used in car anti freeze
 Polymers - aka: plastic
Sodium Polyacrylate - the absorbent gel in baby diapers also used in most commercial hair gels
PEG anything
Heavy Alcohols as they all contribute to dry curly hair.
Ethy alcohol or butyl alcohol etc causes dryness. Whereas, vegetable fatty alcohols are not alcohol as we know it; they are fatty acids.

**Why are they bad for curly hair?**

Silicones are not good for curly hair because it is hard to remove and may cause build up on the scalp.
You'll need a harsh shampoo with loads of SLS to remove silicones but then you are just stripping your hair of its natural oils (sebum) leaving it completely bare bone dry. Then you need a conditioner to restore the softness again. However, most commercial brands contain dimethicone, propylene glycol or cyclomethicone or some type of synthetic polymer. Then we're back to full circle again.

<u>**Suggestions:**</u>

✓ To prevent snagging, breakage and/or frizz use a wide tooth comb or Afro pick and apply a light all natural leave in like Whipped Butter.

If you need to use a brush make sure that it has a wide area & fewer teeth. The Goody Ouch less Brush is brilliant for brushing (in my humble opinion). This will enable the natural oil secretion (sebum) to be evenly distributed from root to tip & the curl remains intact.

**2.** After shampooing - to build volume. Don't wrap your hair like Cleopatra as this will interfere with the bouncy curly coily pattern not to mention contributes to less volume & more frizz. Instead, gently squeeze the excess water from the curls.

If you can, try and get a microfiber towel or one of those Car drying towels (yup that's what I said) they are great for curly, coily, wavy hair.

I think the main thing that we can do for ourselves, is really investigate what is in our products, our lotions, our hair shampoos and conditioners, our moisturizers, etc. We have to read between the lines. If you don't understand it, then look it up! Our biggest organ (skin) absorbs 60% of whatever we choose to put on it. That's why the nicotine patches work, because you put it on your skin and then it is sucked into your bloodstream, or how about the birth control patch, same thing. Now since I have decided to wear my natural hair, I appreciate it so much, (minus the hair dye). But I did realize how my hair feels so much better, so I started looking up what perms do to the hair.

### Girl, you need a perm!

How many times have **African**-American
women been told this? I was fortunate that I
wasn't forced to get a perm until about the
age of 12. My younger aunt told me she was
going to take me to the beauty shop to get a
perm. When I got home from school, I was
so excited that I ran in the house and told my
older aunt, "Aunt Roe, Aunt Nat is taking
me to get a perm!" Aunt Roe immediately
ran and got her shampoo and washed my
hair. I didn't know why, I just figured this
was what I had to do before I get my perm.

Aunt Nat came to take me to the beauty
shop. When she saw my head was wet, she
panicked, "What happened to your hair?"
she said, "Aunt Roe washed it." I said. Aunt
Nat looked disappointed, but we still went to
the beauty shop. The beautician told me she
couldn't perm my hair, because it was
recently washed, so she pressed my hair. At
that time I really didn't care that I didn't get
the perm, because when she pressed my hair,
it was so beautiful and thick!

About two weeks later, Aunt Nat took me
to get my perm. It was nice, but I don't
remember having that thickness I had when
it was pressed. My hair had lots of body and
I could shake it, but it definitely wasn't as
thick. I realized later, after my hair began
breaking, why Aunt Roe was trying to stop
me from getting a perm. I still wonder to this

day if I had never gone back to the shop, would I have ever gotten a perm.

The positive thing about perms is that they are easy to manage, easy to style, and some people really don't experience significant damage. The negatives are, Chemicals damage and the excessive breakage that occurs with majority of afro American women, and the good hair, bad hair theory... I will admit, perms are super easy to deal with verses kinky hair. For the record, I sometimes like to wear my hair straight, and when I do now, I will get it pressed. I am grateful that I have many options as to styling my hair. The thing is, perm is short for permanent. Once you have a perm, there is no going back unless you are prepared to play the waiting game, which most women do not do. As stated above, if 60% of what we put on our body is absorbed in our skin, then that means every time we retouch our perm, additional chemicals are induced in our bloodstream through the pores of our scalps. Of special concern is the practice of parents of little girls, who at the age of as early as 4 years old have their hair chemically processed. In many instances damages occur such as thinning and breaking of the hair.

On a final note, think about how old you are. Then, think about the amount of times you put a perm on your head per year. Then think about the ingredients in a perm. Perms have Ammonium, lye, and petroleum as some of the main ingredients.

Now multiply that by your age, and then take in the fact that 60% of the total has been absorbed into your bloodstream. Do you honestly think that has **No effect** on your health? Perms have also been linked to fibroid tumors.

## Adolescent exposures to cosmetic chemicals of concern

The 20 teens we tested had an average of 13 hormone-altering cosmetics chemicals in their bodies.

Laboratory tests reveal adolescent girls across America are contaminated with chemicals commonly used in cosmetics and body care products. Environmental Working Group (EWG) detected 16 chemicals from 4 chemical families - phthalates, triclosan, parabens, and musks - in blood and urine samples from 20 teen girls aged 14-19. Studies link these chemicals to potential health effects including cancer and hormone disruption. These tests feature first-ever exposure data for parabens in teens, and indicate that young women are widely exposed to this common class of cosmetic

preservatives, with 2 parabens, methylparaben and propylparaben, detected in every single girl tested.

This work represents the first focused look at teen exposures to chemicals of concern in cosmetics, exposures that occur during a period of accelerated development. Adolescence encompasses maturation of the reproductive, immune, blood, and adrenal hormone systems, rapid bone growth associated with the adolescent "growth spurt," shifts in metabolism, and key changes to brain structure and function. Alterations in an array of sex hormones, present in the body at levels as low as one part per billion (ppb), or even one part per trillion (ppt), guide this transformation to adulthood. Emerging research suggests that teens may be particularly sensitive to exposures to trace levels of hormone-disrupting chemicals like the ones targeted in this study, given the cascade of closely interrelated hormonal signals orchestrating the transformation from childhood to adulthood.

## Men and Chemicals

My ex-boyfriend was very handsome with his baldhead. He would close the door every time he shaved, which was almost every other day. I knew he was self-conscious about his hair, or his lack of hair, so I never asked him about why he was bald at such an early age. One day we were lounging in his living room, just talking about stupid things we did when we were younger, and he told me about how he and his best friend would put S-Curls (texturizer) in their hair so they could look like they had "good hair." When his natural hair would begin growing back, he would apply more texturizer. They were both applying additional texturizer every two weeks. They were both putting these S-Curls in their hair, and going to school fooling people into thinking they had "Good Hair." He also said, by time they graduated high school, their hair started falling out at a crazy speed. Now, both he and his best friend sport the "BALD" look. The bald look looks good on both of them, but he really didn't have a choice, and I know that if he did have a choice, he probably wouldn't be bald.

Smoking is also a means by which men and women induce chemicals into their bodies. Smoking causes cancer, heart disease and chronic lung diseases. It kills 120,000 people in the UK every year and is the single most preventable cause of early death in the world. Passive smoking likewise is responsible for several hundred deaths in the UK each year. Cigarette smoke is packed full of roughly 4000 compounds, many of which are toxic and can cause damage to our cells. Some are carcinogenic (cancer-causing).

The three main ingredients of cigarette smoke are:

-- NICOTINE
-- CARBON MONOXIDE
-- TAR

NICOTINE is not carcinogenic. It doesn't cause cancer. But it is a highly addictive and very fast-acting drug. Once inhaled, nicotine reaches the brain in less than 15 seconds. Most smokers are addicted to nicotine and crave cigarettes to feed their addiction. This is the key ingredient that keeps people buying cigarettes and keeps the tobacco companies in business.

CARBON MONOXIDE is a tasteless, odorless poisonous gas. It is taken up by the bloodstream quickly and impairs the smoker's breathing. The gas is also emitted by car exhausts, faulty boilers and fires and is very dangerous in badly ventilated spaces. Inhaling too much carbon monoxide causes coma and death by asphyxiation.

TAR is a substance made up of various chemicals, many of which are known to cause cancer. **Around 70 per cent of the tar in cigarettes is deposited in the smoker's lungs.**

Other harmful chemicals in cigarette smoke include:

-- ACETONE, more commonly used in nail polish remover.

-- AMMONIA, used in the dry cleaning industry

-- ARSENIC, a deadly poison used in pest control and insecticides

-- BENZENE, a cancer-causing agent used in the production of fuel and chemicals

-- CADMIUM, a very poisonous chemical that can cause liver, kidney and brain damage, and is also used in batteries.

-- FORMALDEHYDE, a known carcinogen used to **preserve dead bodies**.

Smoking is also related to causing hair loss in men and women. These are the many reasons to stop smoking.

Another substance that is especially injurious to men is **Phthalates.** Phthalates are a group of plasticizers that add flexibility and longevity to plastics. This is one of the most widespread classes of pollutants due to their wide spread use.
Phthalates are known to *decrease* sperm count and reduce testosterone levels in adult men, they increase abdominal fat in adult men, and they also cause genital deformalities in male babies if their mother is exposed to phthalates while child is in the wound.

There is a more extensive discussion on Phthalates in a later section of this book.

## Basic Skin Care

Healthy, beautiful skin is possible to achieve, but elusive to many. Despite the myriad of advertisements claiming that one cream or one product can give you the smooth, clear, wrinkle-free complexion that most people hope for, skin care is in fact a complex process grounded in real science and human physiology. Many factors contribute to our need for skin care products, so abstaining altogether from them is not healthy for our skin either. Healthy skin begins with a basic knowledge of your skin type, and how to keep it clean, nourished and protected throughout the year. It also requires a consideration of our overall diet and nutritional status.

There are four basic steps to successful skin care: cleansing, toning, moisturizing and use of non-damaging make-up. Our skin types are genetically determined, but can vary depending on the following factors:

- ✓ diet
- ✓ environment, such as climate changes and pollution
- ✓ stress and anxiety
- ✓ cosmetics and skin care products

- ✓ illness or trauma

- ✓ hormone levels, such as during puberty, pregnancy or menopause

- ✓ exercise

- ✓ age

- ✓ degree and length of sun exposure

To determine your overall skin type, use this simple blot test: press one ply of a dry tissue onto your face for ten seconds, then remove it and examine the results. Balanced skin is damp with no traces of oil. Dry skin has no oil or moisture residue on the tissue. Oily skin leaves oil and possibly dirt traces on the tissue. Combination skin leaves oil and dry marks on the tissue.

**Dry Skin**

Dry Skin is characterized by:

- ✓ dry, flaky patches and is easily chapped

- ✓ feels tight across the forehead, cheeks and chin

- ✓ itchy and easily irritated

- ✓ sensitive

- ✓ bruises easily

- ✓ can appear powdery or scaly
- ✓ prone to fine lines and wrinkles

Dry skin is a result of decreased sebum production, the skin's indigenous oil, which is important in keeping the skin moist and lubricated. Consequently, this skin type has less of an oily barrier, allowing water to evaporate easily through the skin. This process can be worsened by detergents, heating or air conditioning, pollution, inadequate skin care, certain chemical ingredients in cosmetic products, overexposure to sun and wind and overuse of soaps and alcohol-based products.

Helping to 'restore' dry skin involves protecting the skin with creamy, oil-based products and avoiding harsh soaps, scrubs or products which contain alcohol.

**Oily Skin**

Oily skin is characterized by:

- ✓ overall shine
- ✓ enlarged pores
- ✓ coarse texture

✓ acne spots and comedones (blackheads)

✓ sallow complexion

✓ tendency to repel and run make-up

✓ resistance to fine lines and wrinkles

Oily skin is the result of excessive secretions of sebum. It can be exacerbated by poor health, or a diet high in saturated fats and sugar. Emotional upset or stress can also trigger more sebum deposits on the skin. Oily skin is worsened by hormone level fluctuations, alcohol-based products and harsh soaps, both of which dry out the skin, thereby activating the oil glands to produce more sebum. Comedogenic ingredients, such as mineral oil and other ingredients which are derivatives of petroleum block pores and can lead to acne spots.

Regular cleansing aids in the removal of bacteria and waxy oils from the pores. Oily skin responds well to alcohol-free toner and a lightweight, natural moisturizer.


**Balanced Skin**

Balanced skin type is rare, and is characterized by:

- ✓ a creamy color

- ✓ thickness

- ✓ smoothness

- ✓ firmness

- ✓ few irregularities or blemishes

- ✓ an even distribution of the skin's natural oil

- ✓ dryness with age

Balanced skin is worsened by many of the same factors which can afflict other skin types.

**Combination Skin**

Most people have combination skin, with oily areas focused around the forehead, nose, cheeks and chin. Other areas of the face can at the same time be very dry.

**Sensitive Skin**

Sensitive skin is not a skin type, but rather a skin condition which has developed from a skin type. Anyone can develop sensitive skin, often due to hormonal changes caused by menopause or pregnancy. This condition can also develop from allergies to cosmetic ingredients, foods or environmental factors. Many ingredients made from animal products, petroleum or synthetics are known allergens for the skin.

The characteristics of sensitive skin condition are:

- ✓ blotchy skin

- ✓ broken capillaries

- ✓ high cheek color

- ✓ itchy, easily irritated skin

- ✓ chaps and burns easily

- ✓ prone to break-outs and rashes

This condition is caused by ordinary soap, synthetic, animal or petroleum-derived ingredients, astringents, harsh exfoliants or drying masks, extreme temperatures and climate changes worsen this condition. Use only mild, soothing formulations on sensitive skin. If an adverse reaction occurs to any product, such as a burning feeling, discontinue its use immediately.

## Climate Change and Skin Care

Healthy skin is slightly acidic, due to the acid mantle, which covers it. The acid mantle is a combination of sebum and perspiration designed to protect the skin from the environment. Each day we lose 850 ml of water through perspiration, so drinking water is helpful to replace this lost fluid. During the summer, water loss is more rapid, and humid conditions accelerate water loss through the skin as the body attempts to cool itself. As a result, sebum production increases, collecting on the skin and clogging pores. For many, this process results in breakouts, so regular cleansing with a mild soap is recommended.

A good skin care regimen during the summer months is the following:

Cleansing with a natural soap, such as chamomile & calendula or soaps that contain lavender.

Exfoliate your skin

Hydrate your skin

Moisturize your skin

Keep lips protected and moisturized

Cover up to with a wide brimmed hat, wear sun blocker and long and loose fitting clothing to reduce the amount of exposure to the sun. Also it should be noted that ninety percent of skin cancers are due to sun damage.

Skin is exposed to very dry environments during the winter months. Heated homes and offices, wind and extreme temperatures increase the amount of moisture lost through the skin. Dry, chapped and flaky skin and lips are not uncommon during this season and are symptoms of unprotected skin. During the winter months skin needs more protection and lubrication to inhibit moisture loss.

Any skin care discourse which does not include a discussion of nutrition is lacking a fundamental principle of healthy skin care. Good health and beauty are synonymous. For instance, a clogged and spotty complexion can be linked to a diet high in saturated fats and sugar. Sensitive skin may become worsened by poor digestion or inadequate absorption of nutrients. Dry flaky skin may reflect a diet low in fatty acids or vitamin E. Skin that does not heal quickly may be low in vitamins A, B6, C or zinc.

A healthy, varied diet helps the skin defend itself against infection, cell damage and premature aging. Increasing your daily intake of fresh, raw vegetables and fruits add vitamins, antioxidants and water to your diet, all essential elements for healthy, glowing skin.

Beautiful, radiant skin is within everyone's reach. Knowledge of your skin type and how to care for your skin all year round, using all natural cosmetics, combined with a diet rich in fresh, wholesome foods will help you achieve the skin you have always wanted.

### Natural Beauty: What is it really?

Natural beauty is the ideal many people strive to achieve when they purchase make-up, creams, shampoos and other forms of cosmetics. But what really constitutes natural beauty, and how can it be achieved?

Many consumers, in an attempt to cleanse, tone, moisturize, modify, shine, color, enhance and so on, have overloaded their skin and their cabinets with too many needless products. Experts have found that 63 percent of all women complain of having developed 'sensitive skin', and many of these complaints can be traced back to an overcomplicated skin care regimen (*Fairley, 2001*). In contrast, the needs of human skin are simple. They are cleansing, moisture, nourishment and protection. Skin which suffers from burning, reddening, pimples, rashes and other symptoms similar to these may be caused by or made worse from adverse reactions to the cosmetic products overloading many women's cabinets. Often many of these products claim to alleviate or eliminate the very symptoms they are causing (*Begoun, 1991*).

When selecting skin care, it is best to choose a product formulated for your skin type. Everyone's skin is individual and varied, but to assist in product selection, and in understanding what your own skin needs, the following skin types have been generalized as in an earlier section of this book.

- ✓ Balanced, which is neither oily nor dry, and similar to the skin type of children.

- ✓ Oily

- ✓ Dry

- ✓ Sensitive, which is a condition involving reddening, burning or rashes when a cosmetic is applied.

- ✓ Problem, which is prone to acne and breakouts.

- ✓ Combination (the most common type of skin), contains oily and dry patches.

Beautiful skin can be obtained by making good choices for your skin, such as using cosmetic products and make-up, which are truly natural. Eating a diet rich in vegetables, fruit, water and healthy oils (*such as polyunsaturated fats, essential fatty acids found in flax seed oil, olive oil, etc.*) all assist in achieving and maintaining healthy skin. Lastly, adequate rest, sleep and exercise also contribute significantly to beautiful skin.

Simple Skin Care Steps:

✓ Gentle cleansing - depending on your skin type or preference: choose a natural soap.

✓ Toning - use a toner which is alcohol-free, infused with essential oils

✓ Daytime moisturizing - light or rich skin moisturizer

✓ Nighttime moisturizing - use facial oils formulated with essential oils

Essentials of make-up: Choose make-up, which is made with all natural ingredients and colors, regardless of one's age. All faces look fresh and naturally beautiful when colors, which reflect the earth's vibrant range of hues, are applied. Rainbow-like colors or deep, dramatic shades cannot be obtained naturally in make-up without synthetically derived colors. These colors rarely look natural, are often trendy and go out of style quickly.

Great looking skin does not mean flawless, masked skin. Rather, lets reconstruct our notions of what constitutes 'beautiful skin' and 'beautiful faces', because perfection does not exist in the natural world, nor does it exist in human beings. Computers, cameras, lighting and other sophisticated technologies create "flawlessness", to create an ideal image no one can attain. Instead, beautiful skin and natural beauty is skin that is free from harmful chemicals, hydrated from within and on the surface, fed with balanced nutrition and wise food choices, and regulated with reasonable exercise. A positive outlook on life and an optimistic perspective also contribute to natural beauty, inside and out.

### What are Carcinogens?
**carcinogens** are substances that are capable of **causing cancer** in **humans** and animals. If a substance is known to promote or aggravate cancer, but not necessarily cause cancer, it may also be called a carcinogen.

# Hair Colors and more Chemicals

Sixty percent of what you apply to your skin gets absorbed into you body, so bearing in mind the huge lists of toxic ingredients on the back of some of the products, if you already have an **autoimmune disease**, you will not be doing yourself any favors. Even if you are perfectly well, chances are you won't be for long if you continue using the products containing the alarming list of ingredients in this section.

These chemicals are immune system disruptors. They gradually invade cells causing cancer and other major illnesses. The use of hair colorants is a major concern due to the amount of time colorant is left on the hair. Our scalp, which is like a sponge, soaks up the toxins in these hair colors. It is recommended that a large dose of anti-oxidants are taken prior to and for a few days after hair coloring, together with plenty of fiber. You should also drink *loads* of water to flush out your system.

A better alternative is to use more **Natural hair colorants** to minimize many of the risks. Few hair colors are completely free of toxic ingredients and those that are, are often not the colors we want. **Naturtint, Herbatint and Tints of Nature** cut down on many of the more suspect ingredients.

However, you should still flush out your system with water before during and after their use. Try to limit the use of hair colors to 6-8 weeks and just re touch the roots rather than a whole head application. Highlights and low lights are also safer.

Many of the products listed disrupt the immune system and the endocrine system. Many people are eventually becoming very ill due to absorbing chemicals from products we use at an alarming rate. Since we use these products every day, often more than once a day,at worst, these chemicals are causing cancer, all in the name of beauty. You can buy organic and 100 per cent natural products that are safe and you will notice the difference on your skin, hair, and health, when you use them. *All products used on the human body should have health warnings on them as in the case of cigarettes!*

Although beauty products don't come with warnings, it is important to check the list of ingredients to determine if it contains any of the chemicals on the list that follows. The list is endless, in fact there are over 800 chemicals in beauty products, many of which are potentially carcinogenic. Here is a list of the most commonly used chemicals in most grooming and beauty products:

### Alcohol (Isopropyl)

This is a solvent and is found in hair colorants, body lotion, hand lotion, after shave, perfume and fragrance. It is also used in anti-freeze. It can cause depression, headaches, dizziness, nausea, vomiting. The fatal dose if taken internally is only one ounce.

### DEA(dienthanolamine)
### MEA(monoethanolamine)
### TEA(methanolamine)

DEA and MEA are usually listed *after* another product such as lauramide DEA. They are carcinogenic and hormone disruptors. Used repeatedly, they can cause liver and kidney cancer. They are usually in products like bubble bath, hand wash, shampoos, soaps and cleansers, shower gels and body washes, basically anything that foams.

### Fragrances

Most beauty products contain fragrance and this includes shampoo, conditioners, facial skincare products, soap, bath products sunscreen, in fact the list is endless and up to

4000 chemicals can be involved. Many of the properties in fragrance are potentially carcinogenic and toxic and can affect the central nervous system causing dizziness, vomiting, nausea amongst many others. On one occasion I was sprayed by an assistant in the beauty hall of a department store. The fragrance made me so ill I had a migraine for 3 days, so I can quite understand this.

**Polyethelene glycol (PEG)**

Unfortunately this can be found in facial cleansers and is added to dissolve the oil and grease *on our skin* It also thickens the product to make it creamy. This product can also be found in oven cleaners. They disrupt the immune system by stripping our skin of it's natural moisture and are also potentially carcinogenic.

**Propylene glycol (PG)**

This product is found in haircare products, cosmetics, after shave, deoderants, mouthwashes, toothpaste, It is also used in processing our food. It is the **active ingredient in anti freeze** and industrial workers handling this product have to wear gloves and even eye protection because of it's toxicity to the skin, yet it is in a high concentration in products we are using on our skin daily and even putting into our mouth (toothpaste and mouthwash). It also has to be disposed of at hazardous waste sites.

### Sodium lauryl sulphate or also sodium *laureth* (SLS)

This product is in 90 per cent of all shampoos and really anything that foams. It is a surfactant and is also used in detergents. Research has shown it is damaging to the immune system, the eyes and skin and when combined with other chemicals in products can also be carcinogenic. It is now seen as a real health threat because it is present in products that are innocently used daily. Problem is, it's residue stays in the body where it then wreaks havoc. Because it gets absorbed by the skin, it is even more dangerous than eating it.

### Mineral oil

Using this is like putting a seal over your skin, or wrapping it in plastic cling film. Think on this one....we put it all over our babies! It acts like a seal and stops the skin from breathing disrupting our natural immune barrier. It stops the skin from eliminating toxins causing them to accumulate. This contributes to acne and by its very nature in causing toxin build up, causes premature aging of the skin.

**Dioxin**

This product is carcinogenic and **500,000** times more deadly than DDT Ethyl Alcohol

**DMDM Hydantoin and Urea**

These preservatives actually release **formaldehyde** into our bodies which is carcinogenic. **Even funeral directors are saying that they only need to use half the formaldehyde that they once used because of the high concentration in our bodies at the time of death.**

**Methlyparaben and propylparaben**

Parabens are dangerous....period!

Parabens are used as preservatives in cosmetics and there are four main parabens in use: methylparaben, ethylparaben, propylparaben and butylparaben. You have no doubt seen them on the ingredients list of many products in your bathroom cabinet.

In the EU, cosmetic ingredients are listed by law so it is really easy to check before you buy. These ingredients are also oestrogenic. That means they have the ability to mimic estrogen in the female body meaning? Parabens have been found in most breast tumors, so what does that tell you? They can cause an escalation in progression and size of tumor. These preservatives are absorbed into the body and disrupt enzyme and endocrine activity. They are potentially lethal and carcinogenic.

**Carmine**

This is in lipsticks, blushers and eye shadows. And has been **connected** to **heart problems**

**Methylisothiazolinone**

This is a preservative with the potential to cause skin reactions and allergies irritation.

**Paraffin**

Used in moisturizers, eyebrow pencils, wax hair removers and much more (See also mineral oil) derived from **petroleum or coal.**

## Petrolatum

This cheap ingredient, once again derived from petroleum and causing the same problems as mineral oil, sits on the skin affecting the skin's natural moisture barrier.

## Stearalkonium chloride

This chemical is used in hair conditioners and creams. It causes allergic reactions and as it is cheap, and also used in fabric softeners, it is easier for companies to use rather than spending the money on plant based ingredients which are deemed expensive, even though the natural products really do boost hair and skin health.

## Synthetic colors

Used to give make up items their color they will appear as FD&C, or D&C followed by number and color. Many of these are potentially carcinogenic.

Please remember **these products *are dangerous.*** They are toxic to our bodies, more so because we are using them daily, sometimes 2 or 3 times. They are causing a build up of free radicals and are causing DNA damage. Many of the large cosmetic houses are still using these products and some of them are brand names that we trust.

When looking for products, first ensure that the products really *are* organic or botanical as many say that they use natural ingredients and in fact do use them but ensure that the "dangerous" chemicals are not in the product. Many products are not 100 per cent natural and indeed it is hard to get them as natural as 100% because some preservatives are necessary. However many companies have an ethos where they are responsible to mankind and the environment and use natural preservatives and ingredients where possible. It is best to find such reputable companies and then stick to their brands so that you really do know what you are getting and that they are committed to providing what they say.

The cosmetics industry is such a money making conglomerate, and large companies know that women will pay *anything* to look good and often don't care what is in the product or how much damage it is causing them. Take botox for example. How can anyone inject botulism into their face? It would be better to have cosmetic surgery maybe? I'm confused.

Also, has anyone considered the potential dangers of spray tanning booths? You are standing in a booth being sprayed from head to toe with chemicals.

There are certain brands I use myself and some of my favorites are: Nubian Heritage, Earth's Nectar, Dr.Bronners, Essential Care, Dr. Hauschka, Jane Iredale and Green People. Although there are many more products to try that are as natural as possible won't harm you.

Green People products are recommended by Kate Moss, Daryl Hannah, Helena Christensen and Davina McCall. Many celebrities are going along the natural route too, so proving we don't need to make sacrifices to look good. Many of Green people products are available in trial sizes and their dietary range is really fantastic for optimum health.

By substantially reducing down the amount of times you are using a product containing chemicals, you are benefiting your skin, hair, body and immune system. I noticed that my facial skin pumped out oil when using products containing chemicals because they are so harsh, but this reduced when using organic products. You are much less prone to irritation of any kind and your skin really looks a lot fresher and younger and glows. When you think about it, how can it glow with chemicals in it? (except in a radio active kind of way, I suppose!!) I Try to make sure that *most* of the products I use are chemical free. There has to be some exceptions though. However I have actually become quite afraid of using products containing chemicals.

Your hair benefits too, and is stronger and shinier. The thing about organic shampoos is that they do not lather as much due to the absence of sodium laureth sulphate, but your hair is still clean afterwards. It may not be "squeaky" clean, but this is usually because it has been stripped of oils. Oily hair tends to be less oily as the chemicals in shampoo are being absorbed into your scalp causing the sebaceous glands to over act. Dry hair benefits because it is not being stripped of all goodness. The organic hair conditioners are fantastic and you know your hair is being nourished. (No silicone in the ingredients)

With cleansers, your skin is not being stripped of its natural moisture barrier or preventing your skin from breathing or eliminating toxins. Bath and shower products are unlikely to cause Candida or irritation as the ingredients are beneficial and not chemical.

Make up is also beneficial to your skin and without blocking pores or stopping skin from breathing. There are many products to choose from and with trial sizes available, (etsy.com) you can mix and match and even take them on holiday. There are also anti aging products and luxurious facial oils so you are not losing out on luxury, just on chemicals and scary ingredients. Body lotions and sun creams are not packed with potentially carcinogenic ingredients and slavering these on will not cause you anxiety about damaging your immune system or sealing your skin off causing problems with toxin elimination.

Also, in a world that is becoming more and more damaged by pollutants and chemicals, you are doing your bit for environmental issues as the bottles and packaging are recyclable. Green people also sell baby products, fluoride and SLS free toothpaste, home care products, sun care products as well as cosmetics, hair care and skincare products. They also do their own body spa range. I particularly recommend their cooling eye gel to reduce puffiness.

Dr Hauschka range is gorgeous with a face care range, eye and lip care products, body care, sun care. I particularly love their light rose day cream as a beautiful scented face cream, their tinted moisturizer, bronzing powder and their translucent bronze concentrate which gives a warm sun kissed glow to the face. None of the products are outrageously over priced and the quality is fantastic.

With so many yummy products to choose from there is bound to be one for you as many organic and natural brands have an extensive range.

### Antibacterials

Overuse of antibacterials can prevent them from effectively fighting disease-causing germs like E. coli and Salmonella enterica. Triclosan, widely used in soaps, toothpastes and deodorants, has been detected in breast milk, and one recent study found that it interferes with testosterone activity in cells. Numerous studies have found that washing with regular soap and warm water is just as effective at killing germs.

### Coal Tar

Coal tar is a known human carcinogen used as an active ingredient in dandruff shampoos and anti-itch creams. Coal-tar-based dyes such as FD&C Blue 1, used in toothpastes, and FD&C Green 3, used in mouthwash, have been found to be carcinogenic in animal studies when injected under skin.

**Diethanolamine** (DEA)

DEA is a possible hormone disruptor, has shown limited evidence of carcinogenicity and depletes the body of choline needed for fetal brain development. DEA can also show up as a contaminant in products containing related chemicals, such as cocamide DEA.

**1,4-Dioxane**

1,4-Dioxane is a known animal carcinogen and a possible human carcinogen that can appear as a contaminant in products containing sodium laureth sulfate and ingredients that include the terms "PEG," "-xynol," "ceteareth," "oleth" and most other ethoxylated "eth" ingredients. The FDA monitors products for the contaminant but has not yet recommended an exposure limit. Manufacturers can remove dioxane through a process called vacuum stripping, but a small amount usually remains. A 2007 survey by the Campaign for Safe Cosmetics found that most children's bath products contain 10 parts per million or less, but an earlier 2001 survey by the FDA found levels in excess of 85 parts per million.

**Formaldehyde**

Formaldehyde has a long list of adverse health effects, including immune-system toxicity, respiratory irritation and cancer in humans. Yet it still turns up in baby bath soap, nail polish, eyelash adhesive and hair dyes as a contaminant or break-down product of diazolidinyl urea, imidazolidinyl urea and quaternium compounds.

**Fragrance**
The catchall term "fragrance" may mask phthalates, which act as endocrine disruptors and may cause obesity and reproductive and developmental harm. Avoid phthalates by selecting essential-oil fragrances instead.

**Lead and Mercury**
Neurotoxic lead may appear in products as a naturally occurring contaminant of hydrated silica, one of the ingredients in toothpaste, and lead acetate is found in some brands of men's hair dye. Brain-damaging mercury, found in the preservative thimerosol, is used in some mascaras.


**Nanoparticles**
Tiny nanoparticles, which may penetrate the skin and damage brain cells, are appearing in an increasing number of cosmetics and sunscreens. Most problematic are zinc oxide and titanium dioxide nanoparticles, used in sunscreens to make them transparent. When possible, look for sunscreens containing particles of these ingredients larger than 100

nanometers. You'll most likely need to call companies to confirm sizes, but a few manufacturers have started advertising their lack of nanoparticle-sized ingredients on labels.

**Parabens**
(methyl-, ethyl-, propyl-, butyl-, isobutyl-)
Parabens, which have weak estrogenic effects, are common preservatives that appear in a wide array of toiletries. A study found that butyl paraben damaged sperm formation in the testes of mice, and a relative, sodium methylparaben, is banned in cosmetics by the E.U. Parabens break down in the body into p-hydroxybenzoic acid, which has estrogenic activity in human breast-cancer cell cultures.

**Petroleum Distillates**
Possible human carcinogens, petroleum distillates are prohibited or restricted for use in cosmetics in the E.U. but are found in several U.S. brands of mascara, foot-odor powder and other products. Look out for the terms "petroleum" or "liquid paraffin."

**P-Phenylenediamine**
Commonly found in hair dyes, this chemical can damage the nervous system, cause lung irritation and cause severe allergic reactions.

It's also listed as 1,4-Benzenediamine; p-Phenyldiamine and 4-Phenylenediamine.

**Hydroquinone**
Found in skin lighteners and facial moisturizers, hydroquinone is neurotoxic and allergenic, and there's limited evidence that it may cause cancer in lab animals. It may also appear as an impurity not listed on ingredients labels.

**I can not overemphasize the need to change your lifestyle dramatically and go organic, or as close as you can to being chemical free.** Basically if you use these products every day, you are setting yourself up for serious health problems, yet so many people are just ignoring the very worrying evidence.

# Phthalates

Phthalates are in lots of products to make them flexible PVC, Cosmetics, pesticides, building maintenance products, lubricants, and personal care goods. These products are plentiful in home, workplace, and hospitals. PVC without additives is a brittle component, requiring large amounts of plasticizers to make them flexible. Phthalates are used to make many products to make them PVC flexible. In fact, 90% of global plasticizer production is in polyvinyl chloride plastic(PVC).

Phthalates are used different ways, but they are horrible for your health. In men, high phthalate levels can cause sluggish sperm and low androgen levels. Guys, if you want to make a baby, leave the cologne in the medicine cabinet, blow out the scented candles, and get rid of that pine tree-shaped air freshener hanging on the rear view mirror. Stop nuking your food in plastic and toss the hair gel. Phthalates literally block androgen receptors, so that male hormones can't plug in and give their male hormone messages to cells. There's a good chance that phthalates also contribute to allergies and eczema in children, and early puberty in girls. In rodent studies, over-exposure in the womb causes reproductive birth defects.

Phthalates are banned in Europe because of certain health effects to lab animals. Phthalates has an alternative called benzoflex plasticizers, and its cost is reduced when it has calcium carbonate filler. If phthalates were banned in the U.S we wouldn't have anything that is plastic because phthalates are plasticizers. We wouldn't have the IV bags that they have in the hospitals. Children wouldn't have plastic toys to play with. There wouldn't be a certain fragrances in perfumes, and nail polish wouldn't last very long. Politicians want to ban phthalates because of all the risk that come along with it, but in some cases the good out weighs the bad.

Phthalates may be a major part of our everyday lives, but if we want to live a healthier life then we need to make drastic changes when it comes to phthalates. If we petitioned our lawmakers or people actually decided to do something about this chemical, then perhaps it will be banned. California and Europe did it, so why the rest of the nation. The U.S senate is trying to make some changes when it comes down to phthalates but they aren't moving fast enough, if people really knew what phthalates were, and all the horrible things that comes along with it, I am certain they would want to make a change in the use of phthalates. Just think, every time your baby is chewing on a teething ring, or you and your favorite perfume, these chemicals are contaminating their little bodies, perhaps slowly developing genital deformities and harming you!

### *Class of phthalates*

Use

Di-ethyl-phthalate **(DEP)**

Personal care products, cosmetics

Butyl benzyl phthalate **(BBP)**

Vinyl tiles, food conveyor belts, artificial leather

Di-*n*-butyl phthalate **(DBP)**

PVC plastics, latex adhesives, cosmetics, personal care products, cellulose plastics, solvent for dyes

Di(2-ethylhexyl)phthalate **(DEHP)**

Building products (wallpaper, wire and cable insulation), car products (vinyl upholstery, car seats), clothing (footwear, raincoats), food packaging, children's products (soft toys, rubber duckies), medical devices

Di-*n*-hexyl-phthalate **(DnHP)**

Tool handles, dish-washer baskets, flooring, vinyl gloves, flea collars, conveyor belts used in food processing

Di-*n*-octyl-phthalate **(DnOP)**

Garden hoses, pool liners, flooring tiles, tarps

Di-isononyl phthalate **(DINP)**

Garden hoses, pool liners, flooring tiles, toys

Di-isodecyl phthalate **(DIDP)**

PVC plastics, PVC wires and cables, artificial leather, toys, pool liner

# Products containing Phthalates

Product Type Examples Phthalates
Automotive PVC auto floor mats DEHP
Auto sheeting L11
PVC underbody DINP
PVC upholstery DEHP
Beauty Aftershaves DEP
Deodorants DBP, DEP
Skin Creams DEP
Hair preparations BBP, DMP, DBP, DEP
Nail polishes DBP
Fragrances DEHP, BBP, DBP, DEP
Powders DEP
Building -Home Adhesives BBP, DHP,
DIOP, DIDP
PVC carpet covers DEHP
Caulks /grouting unspecified
Paint unspecified
PVC drawer liners DEHP, DINP
PVC flooring BBP, DEHP, DBP
PVC furniture covers DEHP
PVC garden hoses DIBP
PVC gaskets BBP, DEHP, DINP, L7-9, L7-
11
PVC inflatable furniture DEHP
PVC inflatable pools DEHP
PVC insulation DEHP
PVC mattress pads DEHP
PVC roofing film DEHP

PVC shades DEHP, DINP
PVC shower curtains DEHP, DBP
PVC tarps DEHP
PVC tubing BBP, DEHP, DINP, L7-11
PVC wall coverings L7-9, DINP, DEHP, DBP
PVC water beds DEHP
PVC-coated fabrics L7-9
PVC-covered cables DEHP, DIDP, L11, L7-11
Consumer PVC aprons DEHP
PVC backpacks DEHP
PVC balls DEHP
PVC bibs DEHP
PVC changing pads DEHP
PVC clothing DEHP, DINP
PVC crib rail teether DINP
PVC diaper pants DEHP
PVC luggage DEHP, DBP
PVC notebook covers DEHP
PVC packaging DEHP
PVC purses DEHP
PVC shoes DIBP, DEHP, DINP
PVC stroller covers DEHP
PVC tablecloths DEHP
PVC toys DEHP, DINP
PVC umbrellas DEHP
PVC weight covers DEHP
Food Packaging PVC squeeze bottles unspecified
PVC packaging unspecified
PVC straws DINP, DEHP
PVC tubing unspecified

Cling Wrap unspecified
Industrial/Agriculture Electric capacitors
DEHP
Fillers unspecified
Pesticides DEHP
Printing ink BBP, DBP
PVC conveyer belts DINP, L7-11
Vacuum pump oil DEHP
Medical PVC blood bags DEHP
PVC catheters DEHP
PVC colostomy bags DEHP
PVC dentures DBP
PVC enteral feeding bags DEHP
PVC gloves DEHP
PVC IV bags DEHP
PVC mattress covers DEHP
PVC oxygen tents DEHP
PVC pillow case covers DEHP
PVC syringes DEHP
PVC tubing DEHP
PVC urine bags DEHP
Pharmaceutical Coating ingredient DBP
Stabilizer DBP
Sources: 4 5 24 49 74 86 98 114 127 144
See the Health Care Without Harm website


So, before you decide to purchase any of these products, look for the ingredients. We need to take more responsibility for our lives, our health, and for goodness sake, our children.

# Recipe Diary

We have provided you with everything you need to make your natural beauty treatments. We also recommend that you create your own recipes from foods you may have at home. It is pretty cool to be able to create a face mask from avocado, or a shampoo made with herbs. The opportunities are endless for what you can create. Usually the foods that are healthy for the inside of your body are good for the outside of your body, with some exceptions.

For example, I don't know if I would use Collard greens on my hair, (never tried it) but nettle is a great herbal tea that is recommended to drink for hair growth, so why not make a Shampoo out of it. If you look on the back of herbal shampoos, you will usually see nettle among other herb supplements. You have an endless supply of ingredients that were put on this earth to simply make you beautiful. Before stores were made, and chemicals were created, we had everything that we needed to be beautiful naturally. My great grandfather used to brush his teeth with salt. He died with all his teeth. When I cut myself, my mom would put Aloe Vera plant on my cut, before Neosporin, and I healed just fine. My mom brushes her teeth with baking soda. My son and I have also started brushing our teeth with baking soda, and all the whitening toothpaste in the world does not match the effects that baking soda has on the teeth.

It is important that you have a clear understanding of what you can and can't use as far as these recipes are concerned. For example, if you are allergic to citrus fruits, then you should not use any recipes that include lemons, oranges, or any other citrus. Even though we have provided you with the beauty regimens that we recommend, we suggest that you check with your doctor if you have any concerns about using the product. It's always better to be safe than sorry. Also, certain essential oils are not good for certain people because of health reasons. Please check into rosemary and sage before you use it.

On that note, we hope you enjoy every beauty recipe in this book. We have provided a blank sheet behind each recipe to assist you if you decide to switch things up. It is good to take notes of your changes made to the recipe so you no exactly what amount of change you added. Enjoy!

All shampoo's and conditioner with items that go in the refrigerator need to be stored in the refrigerator up to a week, depending on expiration date of product used.

Also leave conditioners on head for 20 to 30 minutes. Cover with plastic cap.

*Conditioners*

*All Natural Banana hair conditioner*

2 bananas

½ teaspoon mayonnaise

½ cup honey

Fork

mixing bowl

Electric mixer

Clean squirt bottle

1. Peel Bananas.
2. Mass Bananas in mixing bowl with fork
3. Pour in honey and mayo and mix ingredients with mixer. When it is done you

wont see any banana lumps and mix will be light brown.

4. Pour mix in squirt bottle

*Avocado Milk Conditioner*

½ avocado

½ cup milk

½ teaspoon mayo

Mixing bowl

electric mixer


Mash Avocado, blend milk and mayo in with mashed avocado.

*Mayonnaise, Avocado, Jojoba oil Conditioner*

1 cup mayo

½ avocado

3 teaspoons jojoba oil

Mixing bowl

Electric mixer

Mash up avocado and blend with mayo, once mayo has turned green, add jojoba oil and blend again.

*Coconut Milk Conditioner*

½ can coconut milk

¼ cup olive oil

¼ cup castor oil

½ avocado or banana

Mixing bowl

Electric mixer

Blend coconut milk and avocado in bowl. Slowly pour in olive oil. Blend. Then blend in castor oil.

*Onion Conditioner*

Remove the outer, dry and brown skin of
Onion and not the moist, inner one. Store
them in a brown paper bag each time you
use an onion. When you have about 2½ cups
of lightly packed onion skins, put them into
a pan and add 1 quart of boiling water.
Cover and steep them for 50 minutes; then
strain through a sieve. Leave on hair as for
30 minutes


**Shampoo**


*4 herb shampoo*

For this shampoo you can choose to use 4 of
the herbs listed below

Thyme
Rosemary
Sage
Garlic (dry)
Nettle
Hops
Peppermint
Rosemary

You will also need:

Pot

¼ cup Castile soap
Wood spoon
Tea spoon
Measuring cup
8 ounces of water
Empty shampoo bottle
Stocking for straining

Bring water to a boil. Take one teaspoon of each herb you chose to add, and add to boiling water. Stir. Let boil for 2 minutes, then turn off, cover pot, and let sit for 6 hrs. Put shampoo bottle in sink and put stocking or other thin straining utensil over pot, while pouring herb soaked water in shampoo bottle. Add Castile soap. Shake. Use. (you can also add essential oils such as hops, or peppermint oil.

*Rosemary Shampoo*

10 drops of rosemary oil
1 cup spring water
¾ cup liquid castile soap
Empty shampoo bottle

Mix ingredients in shampoo bottle. Let it soak for 2 days, turning it upside down a few times a day. After 2$^{nd}$ day you can use. Please make sure you shake bottle each use.

*Only Natural Ingredients Shampoo*

Apple cider vinegar
Virgin Unprocessed Coconut oil
Lemon juice
Honey
Tablespoon of baking soda

Dissolve baking soda in water until it makes
a paste. Apply to roots and let sit for 5
minutes. After applying, massage scalp
while baking soda is in it. The sides, back,
middle of head carefully, so you avoid
popping hair from root. After 5 minutes are
up, mix apple cider vinegar with water,
coconut oil and honey, and pour over head.
Let sit for 5 minutes and rinse thoroughly.

## How to Make Soap

Melt 1 pound of glycerin soap base in a double boiler. The temperature should be about 155 degrees F.

Remove from heat and stir in cosmetic-grade coloring. Add 1 tablespoon of essential oil if desired.

Mix well.

Pour into a soap, candle or candy mold. Spray the mold lightly with rubbing alcohol to help prevent bubbles.

Let any bubbles in the soap base rise to the top.

Spray the soap tops with rubbing alcohol to make the bubbles disappear.

Let the soap set up for 2 hours, then put the soap molds in the freezer for 30 minutes. Remove from the freezer and allow the molds to sit for 10 minutes. The soap should pop right out.

## Healing Soap

2 cups glycerin soap base
2 TBLS. St. John's Wort Oil


## Dry Skin Soap

1 cup glycerin soap base
2 TBLS. avocado oil, cocoa butter, almond
oil, or olive oil


## Calamine Soap...anti-itching
Soap(Great for poisin ivy!)

1 cup glycerin soap base
2 TBLS. Calamine Lotion
2 TBLS. Liquid Glycerin
1 TBLS. French White Clay

# Soap with Lye

Shea Butter Soap

Ingredients:

4.8 oz olive oil
4.8 oz coconut oil
3.2 oz shea butter
3.2 oz palm oil

6oz distilled water
2.2oz of lye
.8oz essential oil

Instructions: Follow your basic soap recipe. I melt the Shea Butter in the microwave for about 20 seconds or so it doesn't take long. and I add it along with the other oils.

This recipe will produce 4-6 bars depending on the size of your molds. I think these bars are similar to the liquid soap they sell at bath and body works that has the shea butter in it.

## Honey Almond Soap

Ingredients:
1 cup melted white soap base
1 tablespoon pure, filtered beeswax
1 tablespoon honey
1 tablespoon almond meal
6 drops amaretto (almond) fragrance oil

Instructions:
This is a sweet smelling soap. Melt beeswax in double boiler and hold over hot water. Melt the white soap base separate from the beeswax either in a double boiler or in the microwave. Mix hot, melted soap and melted beeswax. Add honey and stir until dissolved. Allow soap to cool until a thin film covers the top (not too long or soap will

be too cool to pour). Stir in the almond meal and fragrance oil. Pour into prepared molds. Remove from molds when hardened (approximately 2-3 hours).

## Hair Growth Formulas for Thinning Areas

1/2 cup pure vodka

Jalapeño

Lemon seeds

Licorice

Castor oil

Jar

Cut up about 5 slices of jalapeno and grinded up lemon seeds into the vodka. Put mix into refrigerator for 5 days. Take out and add drain vodka out. Add about 4 drops of castor oil. Blend licorice with jalapeno and apply to thinning area of hair. Leave on for an hour, then rinse.

## Iodine Treatment

Iodine

Castor Oil

Simply combine equal parts of ingredients, and apply to thin areas of head. Let it sit and then rinse.

*Castor Oil Treatment*

Castor oil

Olive Oil

Vitamin E oil

Combine ingredients of equal amounts, and apply to thinning areas. After applying, massage scalp vigorously for 20 minutes, then rinse with warm water.

*Onion scrub*

Rub steamed union on your thinning areas for about 20 minutes. Rinse hair in cold water.

*Pepper Treatment*

Grind one tablespoon black pepper and lemon seeds each and prepare a paste using them. Apply this mixture on head and scalp. Keep it for 10-15 minutes and then rinse of using clean cold water. This will prevent hair loss and help in hair growth.

*Honey Vodka*

Russian cure with honey and vodka remedy for hair loss - combine one tablespoon honey with one jigger of vodka and the juice of a medium-size onion; rub mixture into the scalp every night, cover with a cap and shampoo in the morning. Apple cider vinegar used as a hair rinse may stimulate hair growth. Rub vitamin E oil into the scalp nightly.

### Skin blemishes Treatment

½ cup olive oil

¼ cup vinegar

¼ cup water

Mix ingredients, and apply to blemishes.

Rinse with cold water and pat dry

## Lemon Lightener for blemishes

Apply lemon juice to face, let sit about 5 minutes, rinse with warm water.

Olive Oil Facial (for dry skin)

¼ cup olive oil, ¼ cup honey

Blend ingredients until they become one. Apply to your face and neck. Leave on for 15 minutes. Rinse with warm water.

*Skin Mask*

*Sea Salt Scrub/ Yogurt facial (acne skin)*

Fist full of sea salt

1 cup of plain yogurt

Gently scrub face with salt to remove dead skin that may be clogging pores. Salt also kills bacteria, so it will also help in removing impurities in your skin. After you are done scrubbing, apply yogurt to your face. This will help tighten your pores and soften your skin.

*Honey Facials (blackheads)*

Apply warm honey to areas with blackheads. Let it sit for 10 minutes. Rinse with warm water.

*Lemon Juice (large pores)*

Apply lemon juice to face and let sit for up to about 41/2 minutes. Rinse with warm water. Don't leave on longer than asked! It will start feeling uncomfortable.

*Honey Olive Oil Facial*

1 tablespoon honey

1 egg yoke

1 teaspoon olive oil

Blend egg yoke and olive oil until they become one, and then add honey. Blend. Apply to face and let sit for 15 minutes. Rinse with warm water.

*Cucumber Mask*

1 cucumber

½ cup lemon juice

1 teaspoon witch hazel

1 egg white mix until fluffy

Cut skin off cucumber and put cucumber in a food processor. After it is blended, strain with tight knit strainer, have bowl underneath strainer. Put cucumber juice, witch hazel, and lemon juice in the bowl. Add egg white while stirring. Allow to sit on face 15 to 25 minutes. Rinse with warm water.

*Peach Tightening Facial*

1 ripe peach, peeled without seed

1 egg white

Blend together until smooth in a blender. Pat on face. Let sit for 30 minutes, then rinse with cool water.

*Apple Facial*

1 apple cut in 4 pieces with seeds and skin taken out

2 table spoons of honey

Put apples in blender, or food processor and chop. Put apples and honey in a bowl and refrigerate for 10 minutes. Take out and apply to face until it feels sticky. Leave on for 15 to 25 minutes. Rinse with warm water.

*Tomato Facial (for blemishes)*

1 ripe tomato chopped

1 teaspoon of lemon juice

1 tablespoon of instant oatmeal

1 teaspoon of olive oil

Blend everything until it is a thick mixture. Apply to blemished areas. Add more oatmeal if necessary, let sit for 10 minutes. Then scrub off with warm towel.

*Dry Skin Patches*

Place basil leaves dipped in water and apply on affected area.

*Hand and foot Cream*

1 banana

4 tablespoons of honey

3 tablespoons of lemon juice

2 tablespoons of margarine

1 capsule of olive oil

Put ingredients in blender until smooth. Apply to hands and feet. Put thick gloves or socks on hands, and thick socks on feet. Go to bed. Wake up in the morning and take socks and gloves off. Rinse both hands and feet and enjoy the softness.

**Make Your Own Lotion**

¾ cup of scented oil (So Many options! Peach, Mango, Raspberry, etc. )

2 teaspoons of Steric acid

1 teaspoon of liquid glycerin

½ cup spring water

1 teaspoon of emulsifying wax

½ teaspoon borax

Vitamin E

Hand Blender

Funnel

Lotion Bottle

1. Find or purchase a container that will be easy for lotions.

2. Heat up ¾ of the scented oil of your choice, Rosemary, Lilac, whatever your choice is, along with 2 teaspoons of Steric acid, 1 teaspoon of liquid glycerin, 1 teaspoon of Emulsifying Wax in microwave until melted. In separate bowl, with pouring indentation, heat up ½ cup Spring Water if you have it. If not, tap water will do, along with1/2 teaspoon of borax until boiling hot.

3. Take hand blender and as you add oils to the water and borax, blend slowly until mixture cools off. You can also add vitamin E oil and color.

4. When lotion is mixed thoroughly, and smelling like you want it, then pour thru funnel into lotion bottle. Use within a month or two.

5. If the scent is not what you expected, then you can add a pinch more. Just don't add too much!

**Anti Aging**

1 Orange

1 can of Coconut Milk

Peel the skin of orange and allow to sun dry for a few days until hard and crispy. Put dry peel in blender along with about 2 slices of orange. Pour in ¼ milk and blend until smooth. Apply to face, let sit for 10 minutes then rinse with warm water.

*Egg White*

Apply egg white to face and let dry. As it dries, you will feel your face tightening! It is very important that you don't smile or frown while mask is on. Just act like you just got a shot of botox! Rinse with warm water after mask has dried(you will know).

*Coconut*

Organic Coconut milk applied to the face is great for reducing wrinkles. After rinsing with cold water, massage face with Olive oil.

*Organic Coconut oil*- taking 4 teaspoons a day of organic, unrefined coconut oil for a month will dramatically give a youthful appearance to the skin.

*Avocado*

½ Avocado slice

1 egg white

Mash up avocado slice and mix in with egg white. Apply to face and let sit for 10 minutes.

*Almond*

Almonds

Egg white

Grind up almonds very good, then mix in with egg and apply to face. Let sit until tight, then rinse.

Note: You should try all of these mixtures for anti aging before deciding to stick to one. Please practice not moving your facial muscles while mixture is on face. This helps nutrients to soak in skin while face is not wrinkling. Also adding healthy eating habits to your diet and drinking plenty of water is the best way to avoid early aging.

### How to make Lip Gloss

Beeswax or vegetable wax

Honey

Castor Oil

Vitamin E Oil (optional)

Flavoring (vanilla, chocolate, coconut)

Very small jar with lid.

Grade one inch of beeswax/vegetable wax off stick and place in small microwavable bowl. Add 2 teaspoons of castor oil and one teaspoon of honey and a drop or 2 of vitamin E and put in microwave for 25 seconds. Don't boil, just melt. Take out immediately and stir. After stirring, add flavor. Stir ingredients again and add to your jar.(if you need more gloss add more honey, castor oil, or Vitamin E oil.)

You can also add color to this by adding dried herbs, fruit, or mineral pigments.

### *Peppermint Flavored Toothpaste*

Oil of Peppermint

Baking Soda

Hydrogen Peroxide

Mixing Bowl

Measuring Cup

Tablespoon

Pour ½ cup of baking soda in mixing bowl. Add ¼ cup hydrogen peroxide and 1 drop of peppermint oil. Use tablespoon to mix ingredients into paste. Voila!

## *Homemade Foundation*

1 oz dye herb

4 oz oil

1/4 oz yellow beeswax or cocoa butter

infuse the dye herb in the oil for 2 weeks.

heat gently till desired color  is reached.

Strain

melt together in a small NON metal pot and
beat together till cold with a Wooden spoon.
store and use.
Some dye herbs:
 Parsley, Black & blue Malva flowers,
Henna, Indigo,
Sage, Beets, Jamaica flowers, Cinnamon and
Cloves.


## Make Your Own Perfume/Cologne

If you want to make your own perfume, with
your own signature scent then here you go!

100% Vodka, Brandy, Rubbing Alcohol, or
Beer

Essential oils of your choice (mix until you
find the mix you are looking for, also at
health food stores)

Spring water

Coffee filters

Dark bottle (you can go to craft store to purchase essential oils and bottles, if they are not dark than figure a way to make them dark)

Mix about 25% oils with about 80% achohol of your choice, stir well and let it sit in dark for 48 hours or more. (The longer it sits, the stronger it gets)

Add about 2 teaspoons of spring water (more if needed) and blend well, then let sit 48 hours or longer in the dark.

After your 48 hrs are up, pour through coffee filter and into your dark bottle and there you go!

If the smell is not quite like you want, then collect some different smell and try again, you can even collect some flowers. Just play with it until you have the scent made just for you!

P.S. it will be good to go to a Health food, or craft store that specializes in having lots of essential oils so you have a wide variety to choose from, also try mixing oils together.

### *How to Make Sunscreen*

½ cup Rice Bran Oil

½ cup Olive oil or another oil of your choice

1½ teaspoons of usp grade Zinc Oxide powder

¼ Beeswax brick

Heat olive oil, rice bran oil, and grated beeswax over a low flame, stirring the whole time until beeswax is completely melted. Then slowly stirring zinc oxide in. pour in a glass something you can cover. Let it cool, and then use.

### Homemade Deodorants

One of the best natural ways to use baking soda, is using it as a deodorant. It has no smell, and doesn't have aluminums in it. Simply take a damp towel and pat the towel into baking soda, then rub under your arm. If you don't want it to be wet then just apply it dry to the underarm.

## Essential Oil Deodorants

30 to 40 drops of essential oil of your choice (no sage oil for women who are pregnant or have epilepsy)

1 teaspoon of zinc-oxide powder
2/3 cup witch-hazel extract
2 tbsp aloe-vera juice

In a small bowl, stir the zinc-oxide powder into the witch-hazel extract, and add the

Aloe-vera juice and essential oil(s). Fill an 8-oz. dark-glass spray bottle with the fluid.

# Coconut oil Deodorant

/4 cup baking soda

1/4 corn starch

5 tablespoons coconut oil

Combine baking soda and corn starch in a bowl and mix with a fork. Start with about 4 tablespoons/one-fourth cup of coconut oil and add the coconut oil to the baking soda mixture, working into a paste. The deodorant will have somewhat of a play-dough consistency, and will be softer or harder depending on its temperature. You can put the deodorant into a small container with a lid.

## Apple Cider Vinegar Deodorant

Simply spray ACV under the arm for up to 14 hours of freshness.

### Homemade Setting lotion

2 teaspoons of sugar to 2 glasses of boiled water, stir, let cool then in a spray

Also Gelatin is a great setting lotion full of proteins. Simply add 2 tablespoons of gelatin, to 2 cups boiling water, add more if needed.

Fresh lemon juice squeezed on hair is a good setting lotion as well.

### Flaxseed and aloe gel

Add 1/2 cup flaxseed to 2 cups water. Boil water stir in flaxseeds and boil on medium heat until it forms like a gel(about 10 minutes). Strain seeds out while pouring into bowl and add essential oil of your choice for scent (optional) after it cools. You can add aloe vera gel, mix in until you are satisfied(optional). Make sure to strain quickly before it starts getting thick and don't add too much of the essential oil. You can also make a setting lotion with this recipe, just add more water. Or to make stronger hold, add honey. Refrigerate after use.

## Good oils for African American Hair

Jojoba oil
Olive oil
Watermelon oil
Rosemary oil
Vegetable glycerin (mixed w/water for oil sheen)
Coconut oil
**All oils listed should be organic, and in there purest form to work effectively.**

# **<u>Recipe Diary</u>**

_____

_____

_____

_____

_____

_____

_____

_____

_____

_____

_____

_____

_____

_____

_____

_____

_____

_____

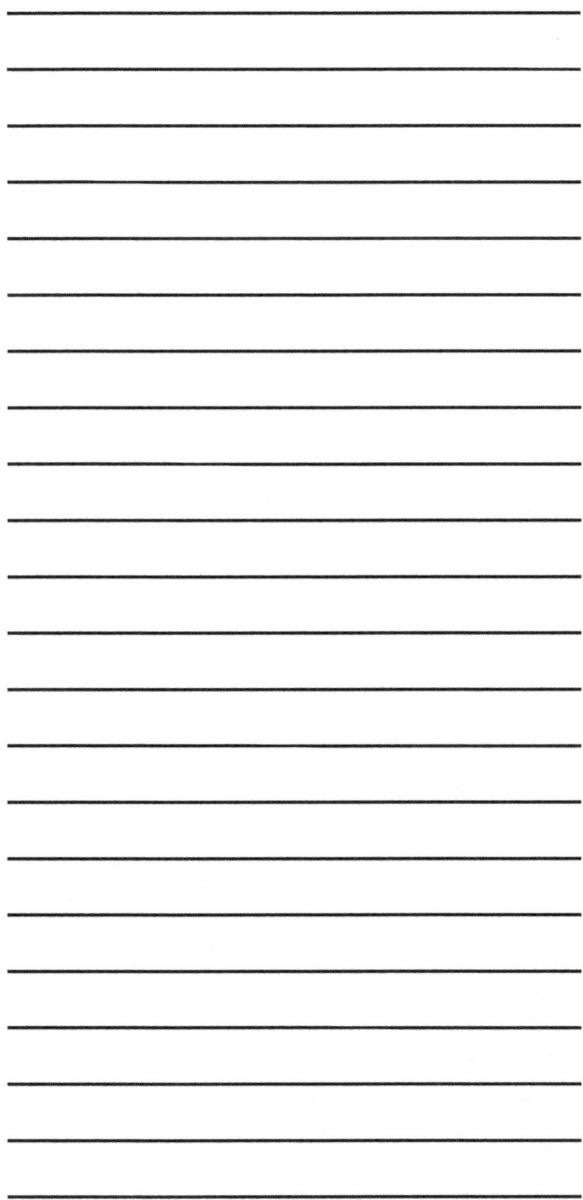

# **<u>Recipe Diary</u>**

_____

_____

_____

_____

_____

_____

_____

_____

_____

_____

_____

_____

_____

_____

_____

_____

_____

_____

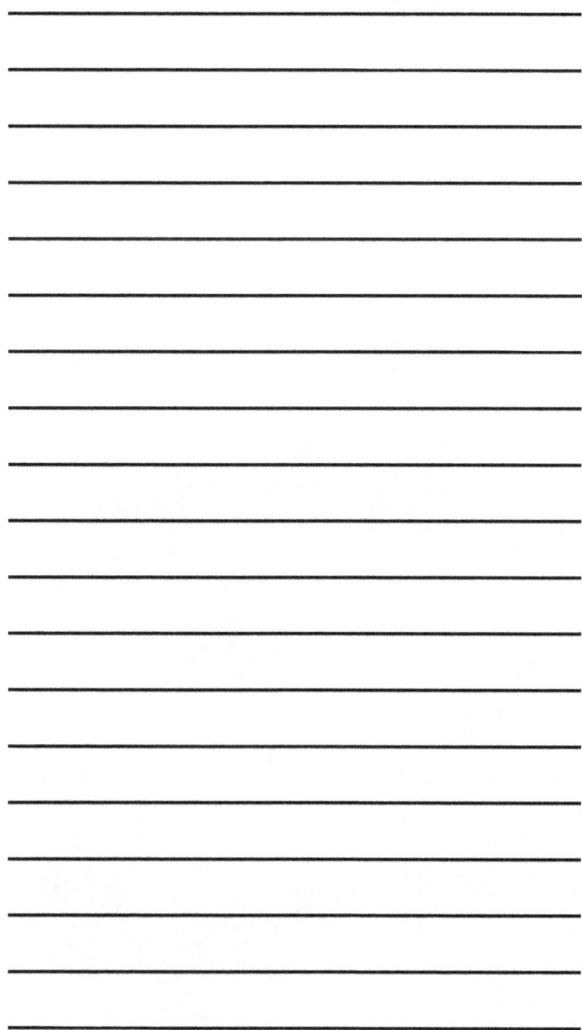

# Recipe Diary

_____

_____

_____

_____

_____

_____

_____

_____

_____

_____

_____

_____

_____

_____

_____

_____

_____

_____

# <u>Recipe Diary</u>

_____

_____

_____

_____

_____

_____

_____

_____

_____

_____

_____

_____

_____

_____

_____

_____

_____

_____

_____

# **<u>Recipe Diary</u>**

_____

_____

_____

_____

_____

_____

_____

_____

_____

_____

_____

_____

_____

_____

_____

_____

_____

_____

# <u>Recipe Diary</u>

_____

_____

_____

_____

_____

_____

_____

_____

_____

_____

_____

_____

_____

_____

_____

_____

_____

_____

# Recipe Diary

_____

_____

_____

_____

_____

_____

_____

_____

_____

_____

_____

_____

_____

_____

_____

_____

_____

_____

# **Recipe Diary**

_____

_____

_____

_____

_____

_____

_____

_____

_____

_____

_____

_____

_____

_____

_____

_____

_____

# <u>Recipe Diary</u>

_____

_____

_____

_____

_____

_____

_____

_____

_____

_____

_____

_____

_____

_____

_____

_____

_____

_____

# Credits

www.ewg.org Thank you for enlightening me on several things that I was totally aware of. I think this is a wonderful website that is very informative, and I hope this book will inspire others the way your site has inspired me.

**Rebecca Sutton, Ph.D.**, Staff Scientist for ewg.org Thank you for your studies. You have provided proof that we all must strive to live a better life free of chemicals.

**Lori Stryker**- The Organic Make-Up Company- It is nice to know that there are companies out there like yours who provide another way to be beautiful without harming our lives in the process. Thanks for the articles you provided. I was astounded to read the harm, and I hope this has the same effect on others. I wish your company continued success.

www.anitagrant.com- also a great website specifically designed for women of color. Thank you for your wonderful information about the kinky curly hair type. You have inspired me!

**Health Care Without Harm** – Your site has provided me with information I never new existed, thank you for the information about phthalates. www.noharm.org

**Well-women.org-Marianne**, what an inspiration you are, I, as well as my Mom have been completely overwhelmed by the information you have provided. Your site is very educational, and thanks you for the explanations about the toxins. I wish you and your family a continuation of great health, pure living, and ever increasing prosperity.

**Stacy Malkan- Campaign for Safe Cosmetics**- Thank you for all the help and very important documents. This is a great site, and I absolutely love what you guys are doing to force the beauty industry to change. Thank you.

Websites I recommend for natural products & make up:

www.anitagrant.com

www.afroangelorganics.com

www.candycoatedinc.com

www.nappturality.com

www.earthsnectarproducts.com

www.theherbalnatureway.com/

www.notjustaprettyface.org/

www.etsy.com


Also, please go to ewg.org and sign up, GET ACTIVE! This is the world we will leave to our children.

Alika Publishing Company will not be responsible for any complications with homemade recipes. Please consult doctor about concerns before using.

# From the author of Chemical Suicide

## www.Alikah.com

Hair Products
Skin Products
Deodorants
Toothpaste
Essential oils
Soaps
Herbal infusions for:
Hair Growth

Herbal Teas for:
Obesity
High blood Pressure
Blood Purifiers
And more!